BEYOND THE STORM: UNRAVELING THE CANCER CODE"

Finding hope and strength in the face of cancer's complexity

by

David L. Brown

Beyond the storm

Table of Contents

INTRODUCTION

In the unrelenting struggle against cancer, our global battleground is distinguished by new research, medical revolutions, and community-driven health initiatives.

Imagine a world where precision medicine, propelled by genomic insights, customizes treatments like never before—offering hope on an individualized basis.

Prevention takes center stage in our plan, with lifestyle empowerment and early screening as our formidable friends. Together, we're authoring a narrative of proactive health and resilience.

Yet, the fight is tough. The complex character of cancer necessitates collaborative solutions, where the convergence of technology, global cooperation, and a

profound grasp of the disease's intricacies shines the way forward.

Join us in this collective mission, where every stride toward progress is a leap toward a cancer-free world. War On Cancer Together We Fight it.

Chapter 1

The history of cancer

There is evidence that cancer has been there for thousands of years, and our knowledge of the disease has considerably advanced throughout this period. An overview of some of the most significant events in the history of cancer is presented below.

Empire of the Romans (second century CE): An imbalance of the body's four humors—blood, phlegm, black bile, and yellow bile—was hypothesized to be a contributing factor in the development of cancer by the physician Galen, who elaborated on Hippocrates' views.

The medical expertise of the Middle Ages remained mostly unchanged during this period, and there were very few improvements made in the study and treatment of cancer.

Enlightenment (the sixteenth century) During the Renaissance period, anatomical studies contributed to a more in-depth comprehension of the human body. However, the humoral theory that was prevalent at the time continued to have an impact on medical thought.

The 17th through 19th centuries saw an increase in the number of autopsies, which resulted in an improvement in anatomical understanding. During this time, several beliefs about the etiology of cancer evolved, including thoughts involving inflammation, irritation, and trauma. Surgical procedures, such as mastectomy for breast cancer, were sometimes undertaken.

19th century: The development of the microscope allowed scientists to view cells in greater detail. During the middle of the 19th century, a German pathologist named Rudolf Virchow put out the hypothesis that cancer came from within cells.

20th century, The discovery of X-rays in the late 19th century and the development of radiation therapy in the early 20th century heralded considerable progress in cancer treatment. Chemotherapy also emerged as a treatment option in the mid-20th century. The understanding of cancer genetics and the function of mutations in driving cancer growth expanded throughout the second part of the century.

Late 20th to 21st century: Advances in molecular biology, genetics, and technology, notably the Human Genome Project, have deepened our understanding of the genetic basis of cancer.

Targeted treatments and immunotherapy have become essential components of cancer treatment.

Early detection approaches, such as mammography and colonoscopy, have improved, leading to better results for some malignancies.

Ongoing research continues to find new insights into the complexity of cancer, and efforts are underway to produce more customized and effective treatments. The history of cancer demonstrates a continuous journey from ancient findings to our contemporary period of sophisticated scientific understanding and treatment choices.

Chapter 2

What is cancer

Cancer is a group of diseases defined by the uncontrolled growth and spread of aberrant cells. These cells can invade and kill surrounding tissues and can also metastasize, meaning they can migrate to other parts of the body through the bloodstream or lymphatic system.

Normal cells in the body follow a strictly regulated process of growth, division, and death. However, in cancer, this regulation breaks down, leading to the creation of a mass of tissue called a tumor. Not all tumors are cancerous; benign tumors do not spread to other parts of the body, while malignant tumors are cancerous and can infect neighboring tissues and metastasize.

Cancer can arise in practically any tissue or organ in the body, and there are many different varieties of cancer,

each with its characteristics, risk factors, and therapeutic techniques. Common risk factors for cancer include genetic factors, exposure to carcinogens (substances that might cause cancer), age, and certain lifestyle factors like smoking, poor food, and lack of physical activity.

Chapter 3

Understanding the significance of cancer gene:

All malignancies are caused by a change in genes or damage to genes. Genes are located in every cell in the body. Genes inside each cell inform it when to grow, work, divide, and die. Genes are bits of DNA contained within chromosomes in all of our cells. When a gene changes or mutates (called a

gene mutation), the instructions it delivers to the cell can hinder it from performing properly. This might induce aberrant development in the body or a medical problem.

Genes work like on-and-off switches inside of our cells. They influence how our cells work by creating proteins, such as antibodies and enzymes, and messengers like as hormones. A gene's proteins supply the instructions to our cells that tell them when to grow, divide, and die (a process called apoptosis). Each gene includes instructions within its DNA that teach a cell how to generate these proteins. When genes act properly, they help safeguard us against cancer. But when there is a change in our DNA or damage to our DNA, a gene might mutate. A mutant gene doesn't act properly because the instructions in its DNA become messed up. This can cause cells that should be resting to divide and proliferate out of control, and this may lead to cancer. Gene mutations can also cause a cell to create too many proteins, aberrant proteins, or not enough proteins.

Gene mutations happen in our cells all the time. Every time a cell divides there is a danger of a mistake being made as the cell makes a copy of its

DNA. Our cells can generally discover these flaws and rectify them before they are passed on to new cells. But sometimes cells can't mend these modifications, and the changes are passed on to new cells. The cells that have a gene mutation due to damaged DNA are the ones that can become malignant. Since gene mutations accumulate over time, we have a larger risk of acquiring cancer as we become older.

The genesis of cancer is a complicated combination of genetic, environmental, and lifestyle variables. Understanding these causes and risk factors is vital for prevention and early detection.

Chapter 4

Types of cancer

Cancer emerges in numerous forms, each distinguished by the damaged cells and tissues. Here are some common types:

1. Breast Cancer: - Affecting breast cells, this cancer can occur in both men and women.

2. Lung Cancer: - Arising in the lungs, commonly associated with smoking but not limited to smokers.

3. Colorectal Cancer: - Developing in the colon or rectum, it comprises colon and rectal cancers.

4. Prostate Cancer: - Occurring in the prostate, a tiny gland in men that produces seminal fluid.

5. Skin Cancer: - Mainly melanoma, basal cell carcinoma, and squamous cell carcinoma, commonly induced by UV exposure.

6. Leukemia: - Affecting the blood and bone marrow, characterized by abnormal blood cell formation.

7. Lymphoma: - Originating in the lymphatic system, it encompasses Hodgkin lymphoma and non-Hodgkin lymphoma.

8. Ovarian disease: - Emerging in the ovaries, this disease primarily affects women.

9. Pancreatic Cancer: - Developing in the pancreatic, it's generally identified at an advanced stage.

10. Brain Cancer: - A heterogeneous group affecting the brain or spinal cord, including glioblastoma and meningioma.

11. Bladder Cancer: - Emerging in the bladder, it may cause blood in urine and changes in urination.

12. Liver Cancer: - Primarily hepatocellular carcinoma, commonly associated with liver cirrhosis.

13. Thyroid Cancer: - Originating in the thyroid gland, it's usually treatable with early identification.

14. Kidney Cancer: - Arising in the kidneys, with renal cell carcinoma being the most prevalent kind.

15. Esophageal Cancer: - Developing in the esophagus, commonly connected with tobacco and alcohol use.

Chapter 5

Causes and Risk Factors of Cancer

The genesis of cancer is a complicated combination of genetic, environmental, and lifestyle variables. Understanding these causes and risk factors is vital for prevention and early detection. Here are the major contributors:

1. Genetic Factors: - Inherited mutations can raise the risk of some cancers, such as BRCA mutations linked to breast and ovarian cancers.

2. Environmental Exposures: - Exposure to carcinogens like tobacco smoke, asbestos, and some chemicals can boost cancer risk.

3. Lifestyle Choices: - Unhealthy habits, including smoking, excessive alcohol use, poor diet, and lack

of physical activity, contribute to cancer development.

4. Age: - The risk of cancer normally increases with age, as cells accumulate genetic mutations over time.

5 . Immunosuppressant: - Weakened immune systems, whether owing to medical problems or treatments such as organ transplants, may boost cancer risk.

6. Chronic Inflammation: - Persistent inflammation, frequently associated with illnesses like inflammatory bowel disease, can increase the risk of some malignancies.

7. Infectious Agents: - Viruses and bacteria, such as HPV, hepatitis B and C, and Helicobacter pylori, can contribute to cancer development.

8. Hormones: - Hormonal considerations have a role; for instance, chronic exposure to estrogen may increase the risk of breast and uterine malignancies.

9. Radiation Exposure: - Exposure to ionizing radiation, whether from medical treatments or environmental sources, is an established risk factor.

10. Sun Exposure: - Ultraviolet (UV) radiation from the sun is a key risk factor for skin cancers.

11. Family History: - A family history of certain malignancies can indicate a genetic susceptibility, influencing individual risk.

12. Occupational Exposures: - Some vocations entail exposure to carcinogens, potentially increasing the risk of various malignancies.

Understanding these characteristics allows individuals to make informed lifestyle choices, conduct proper screenings, and adopt preventive actions. While not all cancers can be prevented, early identification and risk reduction techniques play crucial roles in improving outcomes and decreasing the effect of this complicated disease

Chapter 6
Inherited and non-inherited cancers:

Some cancers are caused by genetic alterations we are born with and that are inherited from our parents. malignancies that are caused by inherited gene mutations are called inherited or hereditary malignancies. People with inherited gene mutations have a higher risk of acquiring cancer, but it doesn't imply they will acquire cancer. However, persons who have inherited DNA mutations linked to cancer likely to acquire cancer more often and at an earlier age than the rest of the population. Of all cancer instances, only roughly 5% to 10% are caused by inheriting a certain gene mutation. But several types of cancer have been related to heredity including breast and colon cancer in adults and retinoblastoma in youngsters. Other cancers emerge from genetic mutations that happen during our lives. These are non-inherited tumors (sometimes called spontaneous or acquired cancers). They grow from DNA mutations that happen when genes wear out as we get older or when we are exposed to anything around us that causes cancer. Most malignancies are non-inherited. Our bodies are made up of trillions of cells organized to create tissues and organs. Genes inside the nucleus of each cell inform it when to grow, work, divide, and die. Normally, our cells follow these instructions and we stay healthy. But when there is a change in our DNA or harm to it, a gene might mutate. Mutated genes don't act properly because the instructions in their DNA become messed up. This can cause cells that should be resting to divide and develop out of control, which can lead to cancer.

Chapter 7

How cancer starts

When genes act properly, they inform cells when it is the right moment to grow and divide. When cells divide, they make identical copies of themselves. One cell divides into 2 identical cells, then 2 cells divide into 4, and so on. In adults, cells normally grow and divide to make additional cells only when the body needs them, such as to replace aging or damaged cells. But cancer cells are different. Cancer cells have gene changes that convert the cell from a normal cell into a cancer cell. These gene mutations may be inherited, arise over time as we get older and genes wear out, or develop if we are around anything that destroys our DNA, including cigarette smoke, alcohol, or ultraviolet (UV) rays from the sun. A cancer cell doesn't act like a normal cell. It starts to expand and divide out of control instead of dying as it should. They also don't mature as much as normal cells so they stay immature. Although there are many different forms of cancer, they usually start because of cells that are growing abnormally and out of control. Cancer can start in any cell in the body.

How cancer grows

Gene mutations in cancer cells interfere with the regular instructions in a cell and can cause it to grow out of control or not die when it should. A cancer can continue to grow because malignant cells operate differently from normal cells. Cancer cells are different from normal cells because they: • divide out of control • are immature and don't develop into mature cells with specific jobs • avoid the immune system • ignore signals that tell them to stop dividing or to die when they should • don't stick together very well and can spread to other parts of the body through the blood or lymphatic system • grow into and damage tissues and organs As cancer cells divide, a tumor will develop and grow. Cancer cells have the same demands as normal cells. They need a blood supply to carry oxygen and nutrients to develop and thrive. When a tumor is very small, it can easily grow, because it draws oxygen and nutrients from adjacent blood vessels. But as a tumor grows, it needs more blood to supply oxygen and other nutrients to the cancer cells. So cancer cells convey signals for a tumour to build new blood vessels. This is called angiogenesis and it is one of the reasons that tumors grow and get bigger. It also permits cancer cells to get into the circulation and travel more easily to other parts of the body. There is a lot of research that is looking at employing medications that halt blood vessel formation (called angiogenesis inhibitors), causing a tumor to stop growing and even shrink.

Chapter 8

Early Detection and Prevention of Cancer:

Early detection and preventive actions are paramount in the fight against cancer. Here are essential strategies:

1. Regular Screening: - Follow recommended screening guidelines for specific cancers, such as mammograms for breast cancer, Pap smears for cervical cancer, and colonoscopies for colorectal cancer.

2. Self-Exams: - Conduct regular self-exams, such as breast self-exams and skin checks, to discover any odd changes early.

3. Know Your Family History: - Understand your family's cancer history and discuss it with your

healthcare professional. This information can guide individualized screening and preventative measures.

4. Healthy Lifestyle Choices: - Adopt a healthy lifestyle, including a balanced diet, frequent exercise, minimal alcohol usage, and avoiding tobacco products.

5. Sun Protection: - Practice sun safety by applying sunscreen, wearing protective clothing, and avoiding excessive sun exposure to lower the risk of skin cancer.

6. Vaccinations: - Get vaccinated against viruses associated with some malignancies, such as HPV (human papillomavirus) and hepatitis B.

7. Genetic Counseling: - Consider genetic counseling if you have a family history of hereditary malignancies. This can assist analyze and manage your risk.

8. Maintain a Healthy Weight: - Obesity is connected to an increased risk of various malignancies. Strive for a healthy weight through nutrition and activity.

9. Limit Exposure to Carcinogens: - Minimize exposure to environmental and occupational carcinogens, such as asbestos, certain chemicals, and pollution.

10. Regular Health Check-ups: - Schedule routine health check-ups to assess overall health and share any concerns with your healthcare professional.

11. Early Symptom Recognition: - Be alert of potential signs and symptoms of cancer, such as persistent discomfort, changes in bowel or bladder habits, unexplained weight loss, and strange tumors.

12. Cancer Education and Awareness: - Stay informed about cancer prevention and early

detection through educational resources and awareness programs.

By actively engaging in these habits, individuals can take proactive actions to minimize their cancer risk and raise the likelihood of early detection when treatment is often more effective. Early intervention plays a key role in improving outcomes and boosting the quality of life for persons affected by cancer.

Chapter 9

Cancer goes viral

As a tumor gets bigger, cancer cells can spread to adjacent tissues and structures by pushing on normal tissue beside the tumor. Cancer cells also generate enzymes that break down normal cells and tissues as they grow. Cancer that develops into adjacent tissue is called local invasion or invasive cancer. Cancer can also spread from where it first started to other places of the body. This procedure is called metastasis. Cancer cells can metastasize when they break away from the tumor and migrate to a new place in the body through the blood or lymphatic system. Most malignancies tend to spread to certain parts of the body.

This has helped doctors establish staging systems that are used to diagnose tumors based on information about where the cancer is in the body and if it has spread from where it started. Many tumors follow a staging scheme from 1 to 4 that are commonly given in Roman numerals I, II, III, or IV. Knowing how a cancer spreads and where a cancer may spread helps doctors estimate how the cancer will grow. This also helps them plan treatment and deliver appropriate supporting care

Chapter 10

How is cancer treated?

There are various types of cancer treatment. It's typical for a combination of treatments to be employed. You may be offered therapy as part of a clinical trial. Treatments include surgery - a procedure to remove the malignancy is the principal treatment for many forms of cancer radiotherapy — high-energy X-rays are utilized to kill the cancer cells chemotherapy – employs anti-cancer (cytotoxic) chemicals to eliminate cancer cells hormonal therapy - decreases the quantity of hormones in the body or stops hormones from reaching cancer cells targeted therapies - kill cancer cells, mainly by interfering with the cancer's capacity to proliferate stem cell or bone marrow therapies – allow massive dosages of anti-cancer treatment to be provided or are used to give the person a new immune system to combat the malignancy You may also be offered supportive therapy to treat side effects. Supportive treatments include medicines to treat or lessen the risk of infection steroids blood transfusions bone strengthening procedures Some people employ complementary therapies, such as massage or relaxation therapy, as well as conventional medical treatments. Complementary therapies do not promise to treat cancer. However, some people may use them to increase their physical or emotional wellness or to relieve symptoms or negative effects. Always tell your doctor if you are considering utilizing complementary therapy. Although many are safe to use alongside conventional treatment, some may not be acceptable. Clinical trials study new medicines to discover if they are more effective than the current treatments already available. This may involve testing a new drug, studying different ways of carrying out an operation, or a new means of administering treatment. They strive to find the medicines that work best and generate the fewest negative effects. Surgery is one of the main therapies for cancer and can be used for lots of reasons. Surgery can be used to: diagnose cancer eliminate cancer find out how big the disease is and if it has spread to other parts of the body control symptoms of cancer restore sections of the body (for example breast reconstruction) Surgery can cure many malignancies. The sort of surgery you receive depends on the malignancy that is treated. Your doctor or nurse can provide you with particular information regarding your surgery. Radiotherapy Radiotherapy uses high-energy rays to cure disease. It can be delivered both externally and internally.

They are most typically used to treat breast cancer and prostate cancer. The type of hormone treatment offered varies on the type of cancer being treated.

There are various distinct types of hormone therapy. They are commonly given as either tablets or injections. The adverse effects will vary and depend on the individual medicine. General side effects can include weariness, headaches, feeling nauseated, and muscular or joint problems.

Stem cells Stem cells are blood cells at their earliest stage of development. All blood cells arise from stem cells. Bone marrow is a spongy material inside the bones. The bone marrow is where stem cells are created.

There are 2 different types of stem cell transplants:

High-dose treatment with stem cell support allogeneic (donor) stem cell transplants

A transplant employing stem cells (early blood cells) from another person (a donor) is called a donor stem cell transplant. The medical term for this is an allogeneic transplant. It's also sometimes called an allograft or a bone marrow transplant.

A donor stem cell transplant can be used to treat diseases such as lymphoma, myeloma, and leukemia. It's also sometimes used to treat some other illnesses of the bone marrow or immune system.

A donor stem cell transplant aims to replace your bone marrow and immune system with that of a donor. This will provide you a fresh, healthy bone marrow, and an immune system that can attack any leftover cancer cells. High-dose therapies -

High-dose treatment with stem cell support is generally administered after treatment with regular chemotherapy. It's used to eradicate any leftover cancer cells and can boost the chances of treating specific types of malignancies or leukemias.

High-dose treatment with stem cell support entails preserving your stem cells and returning them to you after treatment. This allows you to undergo significantly higher doses of chemotherapy than usual.This procedure is sometimes called autologous stem cell transplant. It is used to treat different malignancies and some forms of leukemias and lymphomas. It can also be used to treat some rare non-cancerous diseases.

Chapter 11

Nutrition and Lifestyle for Cancer Prevention:

Understanding the impact of nutrition and lifestyle choices is crucial in minimizing the risk of cancer. In this part, we investigate actionable options for prevention:

1. Balanced Diet: - Emphasize a diet rich in fruits, vegetables, whole grains, and lean proteins. Limit processed foods, red meat, and high-fat dairy.

2. Maintain a Healthy Weight: - Strive for a healthy weight through a combination of balanced nutrition and regular physical activity. Obesity is connected to an increased risk of various malignancies.

3. Regular Exercise: - Engage in regular physical activity, aiming for at least 150 minutes of moderate-intensity exercise per week. Exercise contributes to general well-being and can lessen cancer risk.

4. Limit Alcohol Consumption: - If you choose to drink, do so in moderation. Excessive alcohol use is related to an enhanced risk of some malignancies.

5. Tobacco-Free Lifestyle: - Avoid tobacco products, including smoking and smokeless tobacco. Tobacco usage is a key contributor to different malignancies.

6. Sun Safety: - Practice sun protection to lower the risk of skin cancer. Use sunscreen, wear protective clothing, and seek shade when required.

7. Hydration: - Stay well hydrated by consuming plenty of water. Proper hydration improves overall health and helps the body function efficiently.

8. Limit Processed and Red Meat: - Reduce the intake of processed meats and restrict the consumption of red meat. Opt for lean protein sources including fish, chicken, and plant-based alternatives.

9. Screening and Early Detection: - Adhere to recommended cancer screenings, as early identification plays a significant role in prevention and effective treatment.

10. Antioxidant-Rich Foods: - Include antioxidant-rich foods in your diet, such as berries, almonds, and leafy greens. Antioxidants help protect cells from harm.

11. Limit Sugar and Refined Carbohydrates:

- Reduce the intake of sugary foods and beverages as well as refined carbs. A balanced, low-sugar diet helps general health.

12. Hygienic Food Handling: - Practice proper food handling and preparation to lower the risk of certain malignancies connected to food borne infections.

By implementing these ideas into daily life, individuals can proactively minimize their risk of cancer and increase general health and well-being. Small, sustainable lifestyle adjustments can have a big impact on long-term health outcomes.

Chapter 12

Conclusion

This eBook intended to shed light on the numerous facets of cancer—from understanding its origins to analyzing treatment choices and the impact on individuals and families. By improving awareness, we empower ourselves to make proactive efforts in prevention and early detection. The strides in cancer research bring optimism for advances in therapy and improved quality of life. Let us unite in the fight against cancer, supporting one another and contributing to the continued efforts to beat this strong foe. Together, we can create a future where the burden of cancer is minimized, and lives are not only lengthened but enriched.